Listening in the Dark

Suzy Harris

Third Place Winner of The Poetry Box Chapbook Prize, 2022

Poems ©2023 Suzy Harris
All rights reserved.

Editing & Book Design: Shawn Aveningo Sanders
Cover Design: Robert R. Sanders
Author Photo: Mike Yonts
Campfire Illustration on p. 22 is by Sandra Gibbons, created especially for "Listening in the Dark" poem

No part of this book may be republished without permission from the author, except in the case of brief quotations embodied in critical essays, epigraphs, reviews and articles, or marketing collateral.

Third Place Winner of The Poetry Box Chapbook Prize, 2022
ISBN: 978-1-956285-29-1
Printed in the United States of America.
Wholesale Distribution via Ingram.

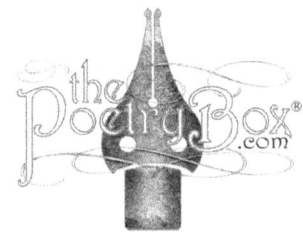

Published by The Poetry Box®, February 2023
Portland, Oregon
ThePoetryBox.com

For my mother, Carla

Contents

Broken Listening	7
Like a Fish	8
First Six Weeks	9
Mother's Lament	10
Mrs. Zaltzstein Brings Cookies	13
Fallibility	14
Whispers	15
Could You Repeat That?	16
Say the Word	17
Book of Night Hours	18
How to Be Deaf	19
Don't Worry about the Storm	20
Somewhere It Is a Snow Day	21
Listening in the Dark	22
Learning to Hear Again	23
Where Poems Are Born	24
Learning to Hear Again, II	25
Language Lessons	26
Lost and Found	27
Symphony at Powell Butte	28
What Is Possible	29
Acknowledgments, Notes, and Gratitudes	31
Praise for *Listening in the Dark*	33
About the Author	35
The Poetry Box® Chapbook Prize	37

Broken Listening

They say people who grow up in two languages
have stronger memories,
 but what of those who grow up with two languages,
  one that is silence?

Memory, then, is like swiss cheese—
 the holes perfectly preserved gaps in memory—
  a necklace without a pendant,
   a story with ellipses.

Before, I heard in the manner of early telephones.
 Hello? Are you there?
  Crackles and static, a few words.
   Then silence.

Now I have new equipment for hearing:
a small rectangle set into my skull,
 a device attached by magnet on the outside—
  but at night, when it comes off,
   silence.

Like a Fish

When I was born, snow covered sidewalks,
piled on top of cars, filled gutters and eaves.

When I was born, my mother told me,
her labor was quick—I was the fifth.

When I was born, my father told me,
he could hold me in the palm of his hand.

When I was born, the world was new,
old wounds held together with filaments of hope,

cars floating on wide wheels
with fins like water creatures,

and I entered this world like a small fish,
swimming up for air, clutching at this new life.

First Six Weeks

no night or day
my first six weeks hums and thrums

nurses coming and going
home is a box called an incubator

as if I am not yet hatched
still in the warming tray

do the nurses hold me?
do I feel their starchy white collars

against my soft cheek?
taste the rubber nipples?

hear beeps and squawks of machines?
do I feel the heat of my father's gaze

through the window where he peers in at me
during visiting hours?

am I really alive?

Mother's Lament

January 1954

1.

At five months, her water breaks.
Did the doctor order bed rest?
She can't remember, couldn't have anyway—
four children under ten to care for and a husband
who needs her to boil his egg, wash his socks,
have a drink with him before dinner.

At seven months, her labor starts.
The baby—*another girl*—in a hurry to be born,
can't wait to turn head first.
Breech, the doctor says, but no time
for a caesarean, and anyway, she is tiny.
The nurse, in her striped uniform,
wipes the slime, weighs the baby
on her scale: *four pounds*.
She goes home a week later,
but the baby stays—incubated—
in the hospital nursery. *Jaundice*,
the doctor says, and the baby is still too small.

2.

The painters are there, painting the living room.
The doctor phones—the transfusion is over,
the baby pinked with new blood, and all is well.
Three of the children are home with the flu.
Only one has gone to school, and *where is she?*
Now, almost dinner, already dark. *Where is she?*
She calls the neighbors, friends, her heart
wild in her chest.

When he comes home,
she sends her husband out with a flashlight,
the neighbors too, searching the school yard,
the playground, the snowy back yards.
The police are called. She stays home with the
sick children, waiting for her daughter.

[. . .]

3.

Hours later, the doorbell rings. Her daughter
stands in the doorway, unharmed.
She says a prayer of thanks,
brushes her daughter's dark bangs from her face,
holds her close.
Her daughter pulls away.
He gave me candy, her daughter says.
And pulls a peppermint from her coat pocket.
Like this. Would you like one?
Only her *this* sounds like *thith*. She has trouble
with her s's.

Dear god, she thinks, *if I can't keep track of
these four, how will I manage one more?*

Mrs. Zaltzstein Brings Cookies

Mandelbrot on a cut-glass plate.
Almond crescents in clouds of powdered sugar.
Slices of strudel jeweled with fat raisins.

She takes sweets across the yard to the mother
of five who looks tired. And for the youngest
who wanders the yard in muddy coveralls,

a gift: a dress like a wedding cake—layers
of crinkly petticoats, puffy sleeves, tiny rosettes.
Years ago, she dressed her own daughter

like a china doll, feared she would break.
Used every waking breath to ward off
tsuris, keep her safe. The children next door

aren't burdened by her memories—
their bicycles left carelessly on the grass,
hand prints on the glass door.

Fallibility

Second grade. We sit eight to a table,
hands folded, headphones on our ears.
We are told to raise our hands at each beep:
Beep. Hands go up. *Beep.* Hands. *Beep.* Hands.

After, my mother takes me to the doctor,
a family friend, a confidant. He has
helped her through the mumps and measles,
chicken pox for the five of us,

stood by my hospital bed
for the blood transfusions
after my early birth, gave us
polio vaccines, tetanus shots.

Always the quick smell of alcohol,
white coat and stethoscope.
Always deep breaths, glass bottles
of green liquid and cotton swabs.

His hands, soft and strong, lift me
to the counter. He puts his cold
silvery watch next to my ear.
Do you hear this? he says.

And this? On the other side.
Yes, I say. *Yes.*
He turns to my mother. *She's fine,*
he says.

Whispers

In those whisper-yellow tendernesses,
I was lost. The street light shadowed
spent clothes on the floor, the chair—
the small candle flame not enough
to see his mouth shaping words.

Even then I could not hear whispers,
and would try to guess, our young bodies
unsure how to find each other
in the dark, our young lives still
learning how to speak, how to listen.

Could You Repeat That?

Could you say that again?

You said what?

Pardon me?

You found what at the store?

You put the gift where?

Sorry, I missed the first word,
the last word, the middle word.

Your name is…?

Wait, you said what?

Sorry, I missed that.

Could you say that again?

Say the Word

Say the word baseball.
Say the word cowboy.
Say the word sidewalk.

In this padded booth,
the only sound is from these speakers.

It could be God talking
and I, the disciple,
leaning close to hear every word.

Say the word hotdog.
Say the word…

so soft now sounds
falter and collapse.

This is me in silence
waiting for the next holy word.

Book of Night Hours

1. Cool sheets against warm skin,
   my arm across your side body,
   palm reading palm in the darkness.

2. Breath in, breath out,
   counting breath,
   feeling heat rise up.

3. Turning one way, then the other,
   feeling the waves of air
   from the fan cooling my warm face.

4. No more thoughts to ruminate,
   just almost asleep quietness,
   feeling the ebb and flow of your breath.

5. More quiet. More turning.
   The thin cotton blanket covers like mulch—
   the organisms below are restless.

6. If I could see, I would see ash falling in the streetlight.
   If I could hear, I would hear the wailing
   of a distant train, the dog's quiet snoring.

How to Be Deaf

Life is an erasure poem where you
try endlessly to find the missing.

Solve for X when you don't know
the other parts of the equation.

Remember Monet with his cataracts,
how he layered paint and color on huge canvasses—
and let what you hear become a poem.

When you feel exhausted by the work
of hearing, bathe in quietness.

Don't Worry about the Storm

Don't worry about the storm.
It's not someone banging to be let in.
It's just the wind, hurling branches at the door.
Weather the storm. Stay the course.

When the wind stops, open the door.
There is silence waiting for you on the door step.
Invite her in.
Let clamor leave by the back door.

Somewhere It Is a Snow Day

It is the hour of hot water
as oats turns to porridge
and darkness lifts from rooftops,
then bare branches—
too warm for snow,
too cold for anything else.

In this hour of blank pages,
dreams tumble out in fragments,
always too many things
and a suitcase too small to hold it all.
(Who travels with a mattress anyway?)

Another name for this hour is
beginning again, or *starting over,*
or *maybe tomorrow.*

Listening in the Dark

Camping by Suttle Lake, walking at dusk,
slathered in something to fend off mosquitos,
we see a giant metal tub on top of a fire grate.
    The tub of an old washing machine, he tells us.
    Chimneys the smoke right up and the light shines through.

Later, in the dark, we admire the now lit up cylinder,
light spilling like thousands of fireflies
onto the faces of children circled around.

Back at our own fire pit, we add logs to the fire,
tell stories in the darkness. This time,
I set the lantern where I can see people's faces,
and my friends, my dear friends, they lean into the light.

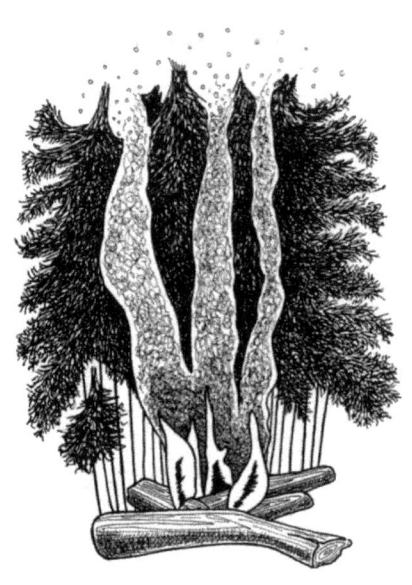

Learning to Hear Again

Snow falls straight and true
covering yards and sidewalks,
while I shelter under a sturdy roof,
warmed by the steady heat of a gas fireplace.

All this, and quiet too,
quiet enough to read aloud
and hear the words echo in my head,
roll around so I can taste their salty-sweetness.

For so many years, I have lost
beginnings and endings, vowels and consonants,
studying faces and gestures
to confirm or deny what might have been said.

In three days, I will be like an infant again,
awash in new sounds, like a toddler
pointing what's this? and what's this?
wanting and needing to know the world,

each sticky, wondrous bit,
each chime and bell and faint clank,
each creaky floorboard,
each soft voice and spoken word.

Tell me, what is the sound of snow falling?
What is the sound branches make
as they bend under the weight of snow?
And do camellias sigh when snow
      covers their scarlet blooms?

Be patient with me. I'm learning.

Where Poems Are Born

In my head, a device sends electrical signals
to my brain. My brain translates these beeps
into words. In this pool of language,

poems are born, raised on the page,
spill out in messy streams of words,
echo in empty chambers until they find

a quiet spot to land. Not a word
alone, but great gushes of words
finding their way home.

Learning to Hear Again, II

The way sound now echoes inside my head—
and all the ticks and taps and dings, unheard before.
Words ring clear and true, but not quite right—
sounds like everyone is talking from the bottom of a well.

All the ticks and taps and dings, unheard before—
some say like chipmunks, robots, or Mickey Mouse.
For me, it's like everyone is talking from the bottom of a well.
Patience and practice, they say. It will get better.

For some, it's like chipmunks, robots or Mickey Mouse.
Not normal, no, but still a wonder to hear again.
Patience and practice, they say. It will get better—
layers of sound unfolding like an *a cappela* choir.

Not normal, no, but still a wonder to hear again.
Words ring clear and true, but not quite right.
Soon, layers of sound will unfold like an *a cappela* choir,
exquisite harmony instead of echoes inside my head.

Language Lessons

First lesson:

> Let it swim and swish.
> Let it travel through time and space.
> Let consonants be crisp.
> Let vowels be smooth and roll like waves.

Second lesson:

> Let dings and ticks and beeps recede.
> Let syllables glove together.
> Let words arrive true and clear.

Third lesson:

> Let the singer's voice rise above.
> Let wind quiet in the trees.
> Let there be café booths for all who desire.

Fourth lesson:

> Gather many pillows and rugs.
> Let softness absorb the hard edges.
> Sit close and listen.

Fifth lesson:

> Ask. Ask again.
> Repeat.

Lost and Found

We say "lost hearing"
like it's something you might find again
in the lost and found.

The survey asks: *are you still as lost*
as you were before? You mean in following conversations? No.

Or do you mean *is my hearing as lost as it was before?*
No, but it's not been found as much as resurrected from the dead.

Or maybe you mean *metaphysically lost*, my spirit floating above
looking for a way to reenter my body? No, I do not feel lost in that way.
My spirit has not left me. I am not lost.

But nor was I lost before, or maybe I was—all those missing words,
and me, grasping for sense in the space between.

Symphony at Powell Butte

I hear wind dance in tall grasses
and earth's slow rotation.
I hear clouds gliding above
and unseen birds chittering in trees.
I hear ancient rocks reminiscing to each other
about when they were part of something bigger.
I hear our dog asking for water
as we climb the last hill,
then earth again in its lurch forward.

What Is Possible

My voice travels so far to be heard.
In this house of quiet, my voice
rattles on to the dog
who sleeps curled into herself
purring under her breath like a cat.

My voice speaks to the teakettle,
which answers with a song,
and to the refrigerator
which answers with a hum I can't hear

and through the wall
to the workers next door
laying plaster over wallboard,
who walk out to the sidewalk
for a smoke and even there

my voice travels, unseen,
seeking other voices. Together,
our voices travel like clouds,
cross borders easily,
falling like rain on dry lands.

Listen, a powerful voice is inside you
and outside you. Each time it rains
remember your voice in the clouds,
mine too, gathering strength.

Acknowledgments, Notes, and Gratitudes

Acknowledgments:

Thank you to the editors of the following journals in which these poems first appeared:

"Could You Repeat That?" and "Say the Word" appeared in a special folio on Disability Poetics for *Tupelo Quarterly*.

"What is Possible," "Learning to Hear Again," "Learning to Hear Again II," and "Symphony at Powell Butte" were first published by *Clackamas Literary Review*.

"Mrs. Zaltzstein Brings Cookies" was first published in *Fireweed: Poetry of Oregon* and is collected in the Indiana State Library's INverse Poetry Archive.

Notes:

"Broken Listening" was inspired by the Lebanese poet Zeina Hashem Beck's "Broken Ghazal: Speak Arabic" ("They say people who grow up in two languages have stronger memories…").

I adapted "Mother's Lament, 1953" from an unpublished short story by my mother, Carla Harris, titled "Little Girl Gone Astray" (1954). Both are based on the true event of my sister Jill's kidnapping at age six shortly after I was born. Carla's story is posted at http://carlaharris20.blogspot.com/p/little-girl-gone-astray.html.

In "How to be Deaf," the reference to Monet was inspired by Lisel Muller's "Monet Refuses the Operation."

[…]

The pantoum "Learning to Hear Again II" emerged from a poetic forms class taught by John Sibley Williams.

"Language Lessons" was inspired by the poem "Mind of My Mind" by Jacqueline Johnson.

"What is Possible" was inspired by a poem of the same name by Adrienne Rich.

In Gratitude:

To my writing partner and friend Vivienne Popperl, and my critique group—Vivienne, Dale Champlin, Kris Demien, and Ann Farley. Your help and support have been invaluable.

To my family—Tom, Ben and Elizabeth Coleman—for always listening and creating safe space for these poems to emerge.

To my surgeon—John Goddard—who made it possible for me to hear again, and the audiologists—Sara Funitake and others who encouraged me to take this leap of faith and helped me all along the way.

Praise for *Listening in the Dark*

I have seldom encountered a series of poems so closely linked and connected as a whole. This chapbook tenderly addresses the poet's lifelong hearing loss with a surprising precision of language, starting at the very beginning of life and reimagining that time of "growing up with two languages,/ One that is silence." No doubt these tender poems will help many readers to feel less alone as they navigate their own worlds of memory, loss, and resilience.

—James Crews, contest judge
poet, editor of *How to Love the World*

This chapbook from Suzy Harris offers us—in richly musical, image-laden lines—a Phoenix- tale. Mostly deaf by her mid 60's, the poet exists in a too-silent world where "sounds/ falter and collapse." Then she undergoes cochlear implants in both ears, artificial devices completely replacing her profoundly faulty natural hearing. With lyric intensity, her poems convey Harris' experiences as she slowly undertakes the eerie process of learning a whole new universe of sound, translating the implants' "ticks and taps and dings" into what's recognizable. Risen from its own ashes, the poet's new sense of hearing leads her toward the "exquisite harmony" of soaring renewal.

—Paulann Petersen, Oregon Poet Laureate Emerita

Listening In the Dark is a visceral prosodic manual of "How to be Deaf," a title of one poem in this triumphant collection of a survivor poet, "…who grows-up with two languages,/ One that is silence?," in which "Life is an erasure poem where you/ try endlessly to find the meaning." Suzy Harris propels us into her world—an exultant quest from "Broken Listening" to the cacophony and wonder of sound. This is a collection of lived experience that only Harris could author.

—Willa Schneberg, LCSW,
recipient of the Oregon Book Award for Poetry;
author of *The Naked Room* (forthcoming)

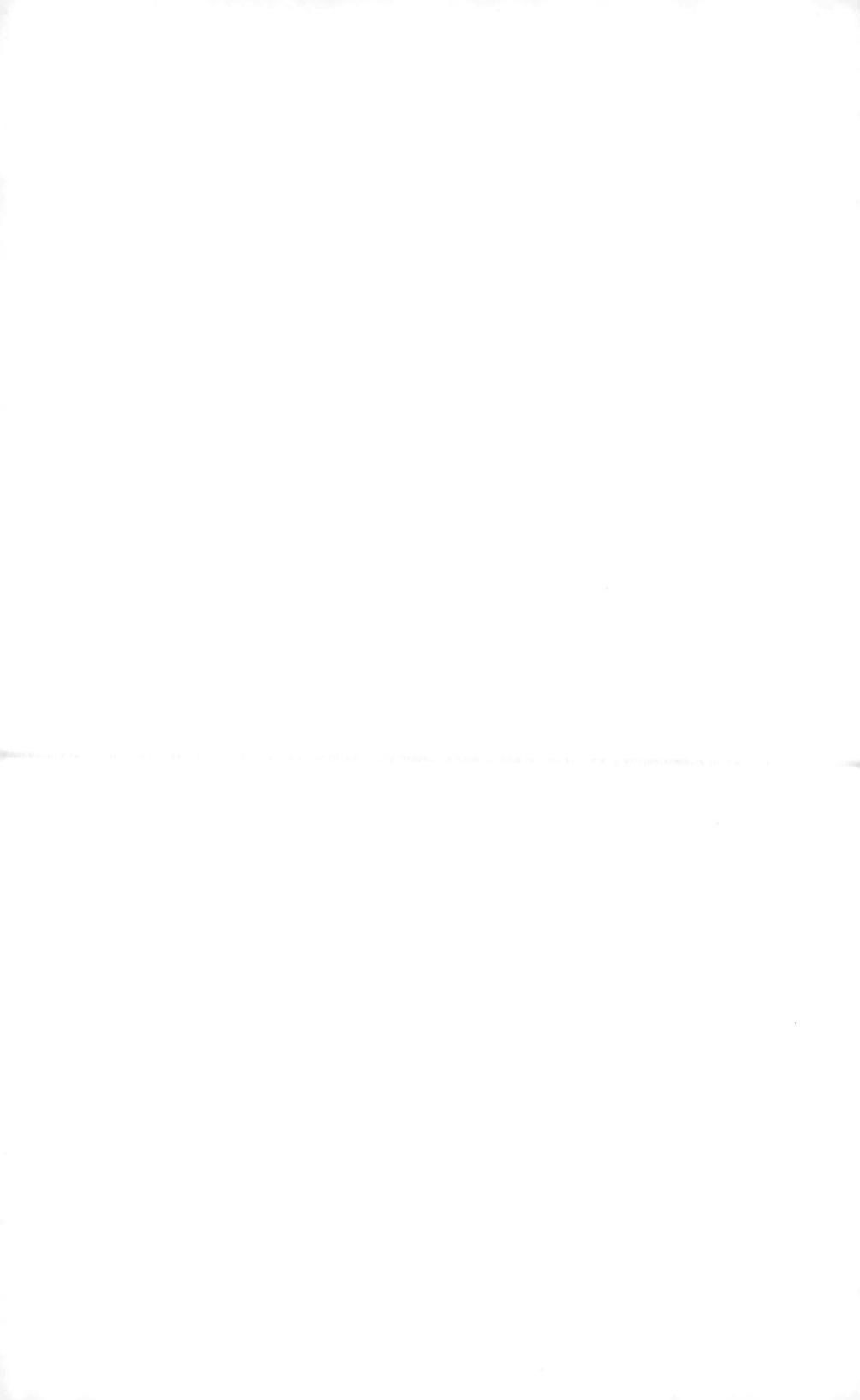

About the Author

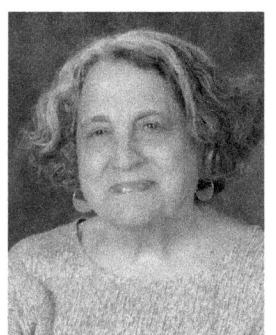

Suzy Harris lives in Portland, Oregon. Her poems have appeared in *Calyx*, *Clackamas Literary Review*, *Switchgrass Review*, *The Poeming Pigeon*, and *Williwaw*, among other journals and anthologies. She has been an Oregon Poetry Association prize winner and recently served as poetry editor of *Timberline Review*.

Suzy is a retired attorney who is learning to hear again with two cochlear implants. Born and raised in Indiana, she is grateful to call the Pacific Northwest home.

The Poetry Box® Chapbook Prize

The Poetry Box® Chapbook Prize is open to both established poets and emerging talent alike. The contest is open to poets residing in the United States and is open for submissions each year during the month of February. Find more information at ThePoetryBox.com.

2022 Winners
Tracking the Fox by Rosalie Sanara Petrouske
Elemental Things by Michael S. Glaser
Listening in the Dark by Suzy Harris

2021 Winners
Erasures of My Coming Out (Letter) by Mary Warren Foulk
Of the Forest by Linda Ferguson
Let's Hear It for the Horses by Tricia Knoll

2020 Winners
The Day of My First Driving Lesson by Tiel Aisha Ansari
My Mother Never Died Before by Marcia B. Loughran
Off Coldwater Canyon by C.W. Emerson

2019 Winners
Moroccan Holiday by Lauren Tivey
Hello, Darling by Christine Higgins
Falling into the River by Debbie Hall

2018 Winners
Shrinking Bones by Judy K. Mosher
November Quilt by Penelope Scambly Schott
14: Antología del Sonoran by Christopher Bogart
Fireweed by Gudrun Bortman

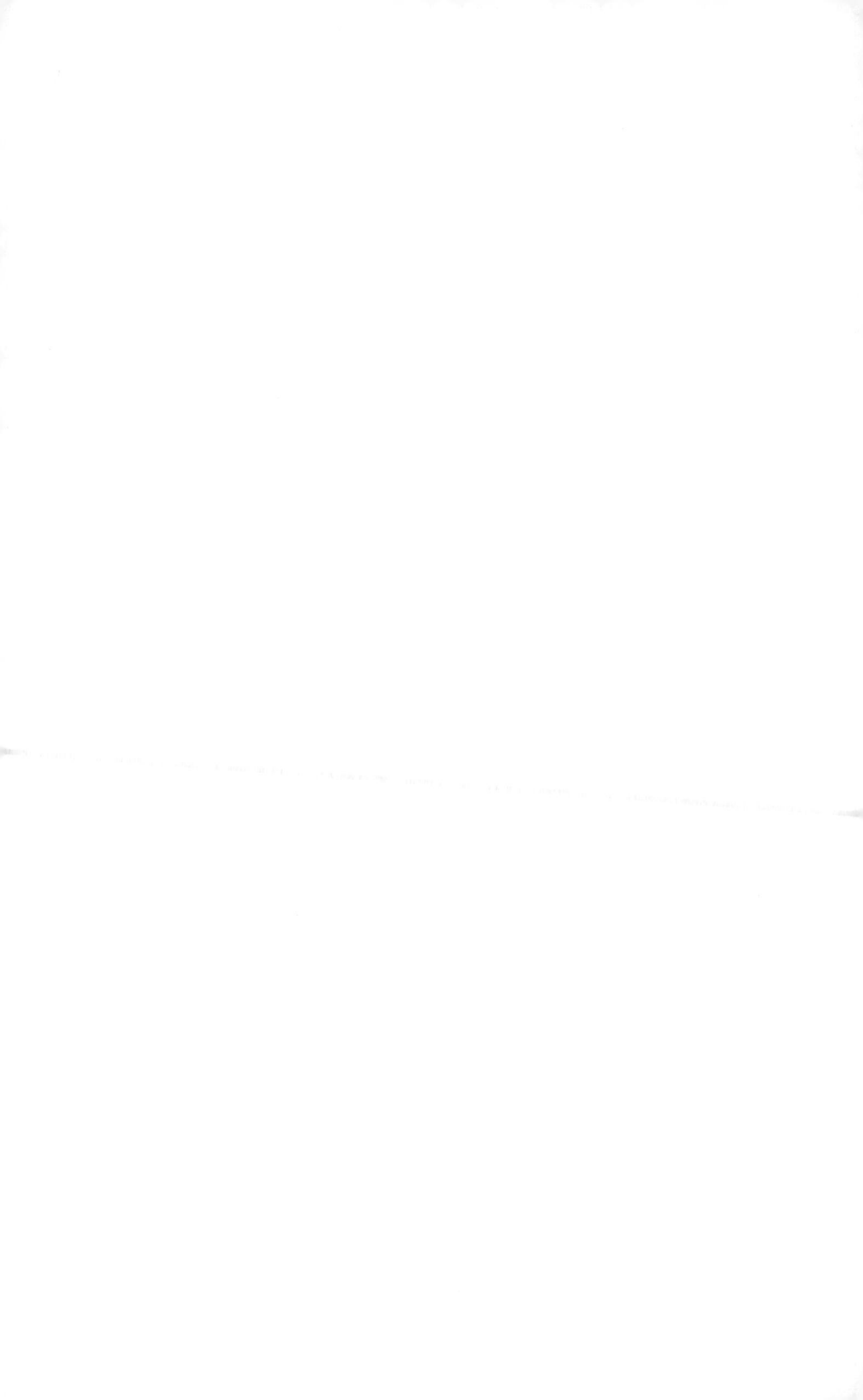

www.ingramcontent.com/pod-product-compliance
Lightning Source LLC
LaVergne TN
LVHW050027080526
838202LV00069B/6953